KETOGENIC DIET

The Low Carb Guide For
Long-Term & Rapid Weight Loss

+ 40 Keto Recipes With Images & Bonus Meal Plan

Table of Contents

Introduction

Welcome, and thank you so much for putting your trust in me by choosing my book to read as your ketogenic diet guide! This book is packed full of helpful tips to help you get started and includes delicious low-carb recipes to keep you on track. Now, there may be a number of reasons you are reading this book. Maybe you are looking to lose weight, have lost weight in the past but just can't seem to keep it off in the long run, or maybe you just want to find a way to cut carbs and live a healthier life. No matter what the reason, this book will be your new go-to guide for a keto way of life.

If you're new to ketogenic dieting, this will be the perfect place for you to start. I encourage you to go through the book chapter by chapter to see how this diet works, how to make the most of it and if this is something you think could work for you. If you're a seasoned ketogenic dieter and are just looking for some new and exciting recipes to incorporate into your diet, feel free to jump straight to the recipe section. This book features forty mouthwatering keto recipes to help make keto taste absolutely delicious.

Again, I thank you for reading my book, and I am so excited for you to start your ketogenic diet journey with me here today!

Example Recipe

Usually, when you're previewing cookbooks on Amazon, you'll just see an introduction or guide instead of what the recipes look like. So I'd like to show you an example of a recipe before we get into the Ketogenic Guide, you'll find it below.

These recipes are Ketogenic and have been developed to be:

- Low-carb – All recipes are all less than 10g net carbs per serving.
- Easy to follow – All recipes have step-by-step instructions with detailed nutritional information.
- Easy on the eyes – All recipes have Images included.

Turkey Lettuce Wrap

If your keto diet has you missing carbs, don't worry because this turkey lettuce wrap closely resembles the gluten loaded wraps you used to enjoy while packing in health benefits instead!

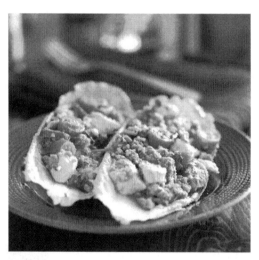

Dietary Label: (GF, DF, EF)
Serves: 4
Prep Time: 15 minutes
Cook Time: 10 minutes

Ingredients:

- 1 lb. of organic ground turkey
- 1 tsp. ground cumin
- 1 tsp. garlic powder
- 1 cup of cherry tomatoes, sliced in half
- 1 cup cubed avocado
- ½ cup of fresh cilantro
- 8 large lettuce leaves for serving
- 1 Tbsp. coconut oil for cooking

Directions:

1. Start by preheating a large skillet over medium heat with the coconut oil. Add in the ground turkey and sauté for about 5-10 minutes or until thoroughly cooked through. Add the cumin, and garlic powder.
2. Next, add in the remaining ingredients, minus the lettuce leaves and gently stir.
3. Add two lettuce leaves per plate, and scoop the turkey mixture onto the lettuce leaf to form a lettuce wrap.
4. Enjoy two wraps per serving!

Serving Suggestions: Serve with a dollop of sour cream or unsweetened plain Greek yogurt for topping.

Substitutions:

- Swap out the cilantro for parsley if desired, and use grass-fed ground beef in place of the turkey if desired.

Nutritional Information:

Carbohydrates: 7g
Net Carbs: 3g
Sugar: 1g
Fiber: 4g
Fats: 11g
Protein: 27g
Calories: 226

How to Use This Book

Part 1: Ketogenic Diet 101

Part 1 of this book is packed full of helpful information to give you everything you ever wanted to know about the ketogenic diet. I have broken down the basics and get straight to business teaching you the basics on this diet so that you can start your ketogenic diet safely, and have fun doing it. I will also talk about who this diet suits best, and how you can reach ketosis, which is what everyone really wants to know! Use this section as your initial guide to navigating the ketogenic dieting waters, so that you can get started on your new way of life.

Part 2: The Easy Way to Get Started

Part 2 of this book is full of information on easy ways to get you started on your ketogenic dieting journey. We will discuss simple tips to help you get started, foods to avoid, foods to stock up on as well as the cutlery and gadgets that will make your life easier.

Part 3: Seamless Ketogenic Dieting

In Part 3, we get down to business and talk about how you can seamlessly start keto eating. We talk about the common ketogenic diet mistakes so that you don't have to worry about making them, as well as some tips on how to avoid those all too well know sugar cravings and how to stop them in their tracks.

Part 4: 7 Day Keto Meal Plan

In this section, I share a 7-day meal plan with recipes from the 40 mouthwatering recipe section of this book. Feel free to swap in any recipe you would like to custom design your own 7-day keto meal plan.

Part 5: 40 Mouthwatering Ketogenic Recipes

Throughout the recipe section of this book, you will notice labels and icons to make reading this book that much easier. The goal of this book is to provide you with straightforward and deliciously easy to read recipes so that you focus your time on making deliciously amazing dishes. You will notice the following labels on the recipes to help you determine if a recipe is suitable for your dietary needs and preferences.

GF: Gluten free
DF: Dairy free
V: Vegan
EF: Egg free
SF: Seafood based

Substitutions:

You will also see a substitution section below each recipe to make a recipe friendly for different dietary preferences. Each recipe will contain a dairy free and egg free substitution recommendation if appropriate for the recipe.

Part 1

Ketogenic Diet 101

Chapter 1

What the Ketogenic Diet is and how it works

"Nothing can bring you peace but yourself."
- Ralph Waldo Emerson

If you're reading this book, you may be asking yourself what the ketogenic diet is? Many of us associate the ketogenic diet to be a low carb way of eating, but there is much more to it than that. We are going to dive into talking about what exactly this diet is, and how it works so that you can get started on your health journey as soon as possible!

First and foremost, the ketogenic diet has been deemed a sure-fire way to lose weight. It has been used as a diet to assist in weight loss for quite some time now and is continuously gaining popularity. What most people don't know, though, is that the ketogenic diet was discovered many, many years ago by a physician named, Dr. Russel Wilder of the Mayo Clinic. This diet has been around for over 92 years and was originally used as the sole treatment for those who suffered from chronic seizures. This was the only approach to treating epilepsy back in the 1920's before medications for this condition came on the market.

In the 1940's when anti-seizure medications came on the market, the ketogenic diet was not as readily used, and people lost interest; however, this diet sparked new interest as of recently, and more research continues to be done every day on the health promoting benefits. Many people are beginning to turn to this diet as a natural way to take control of their health as opposed to using pharmaceutical measures.

The basis of this diet is a focus on low-carb eating to allow your body to enter into a state of ketosis and a diet high in fats to keep your energy levels up and to help your body turn into a fat burning machine. The amazing thing about the ketogenic diet is that this diet does only assist those who are looking to lose weight, but research has shown that this diet is helpful in reducing symptoms associated with conditions such as Alzheimer's disease and is still used as a complementary measure to epilepsy treatments. There is certainly something to be said about this diet due to the science that has back its health promoting benefits for so many years, and may be the hidden secret to reducing the obesity epidemic as well.

So, how does this diet work exactly? When you follow a ketogenic diet, you cut your carbs enough, so your body begins to burn fat for fuel instead of carbohydrates. This causes your body to go into a state of ketosis and allows for weight loss. In the following chapters, we are going to speak in depth about how to reach ketosis and more about how this diet works. Head over to the next chapter to determine if the ketogenic diet is the right diet for you.

Chapter 2

Is the Ketogenic Diet for me?

"The mind is everything. What you think you will become."
- Buddha

As with any diet, not all diets work for everyone and certain precautions that need to be taken before starting any new diet plan. Despite the fact that this diet has been shown to drastically assist people in their weight loss goals, and help with various other health conditions this does not mean that the diet is safe for everyone.

To be sure that this diet is safe for you, speak with your physician before getting started. One of the reasons this diet may be deemed as unsafe for some is prescription medications. There are a number of different medications that may be impacted by starting a low carb diet like the keto diet. Certain medications may have a stronger effect on the body during the first few weeks of starting the diet, and certain side effects may be a sudden drop in blood pressure in those taking blood pressure prescription medications, and blood sugar levels may drop to a dangerous level in those taking insulin. The bottom line is always to speak with your doctor before starting this diet to make sure this is a safe option; they may request frequent follow-up visits during the first couple of months to make sure everything is within a safe limit.

Secondly, certain medical conditions warrant specific attention and concern before starting this diet. This diet may not be safe for those with gallbladder disease, or those who have had bariatric surgery. This diet is very high in fat which can cause the potential for issues for anyone suffering from either of those conditions. Those who are pregnant or breastfeeding may also not be candidates to start the ketogenic diet, as there is a high nutritional requirement for both mom and baby that the ketogenic diet would not be able to fulfill. Lastly, those with pancreatic insufficiency, those who suffer from frequent kidney stones, or anyone who suffers from any eating disorder needs to discuss this diet with their doctor before starting. Eating disorders may be problematic because of the intense focus on food, and may not be appropriate. Always check with a doctor first.

The take home message here is that although the ketogenic diet has proven to have numerous health benefits and may be the answer to your weight loss goals as with any diet, it's critical to always check with your physical before starting. If you check with your doctor and get the green light to start, you don't have to worry, and you can start the ketogenic diet without having to worry if this is something that is going to work for you. Always veer on the safe side, your health is too important to take any risks.

Chapter 3
How to achieve Ketosis

"When the world says, "Give up," Hope whispers,
"Try it one more time."
- Unknown

So, now that you know what the ketogenic diet is you likely want to know how exactly you achieve ketosis, and why you want to in the first place.

The first thing to address are ketones, and what they are. Ketone bodies are produced in the body when your body is metabolizing fats. When you are following a ketogenic diet, and your body enters into a state of ketosis, you will have an increase in the amount of ketone bodies in your blood which is evidence that your body is more efficiently burning fat. This is why everyone following a ketogenic diet wants to reach ketosis! A state of ketosis helps with weight loss.

So, how do you reach ketosis? Ketosis occurs when you deprive your body of carbohydrates by significantly restricting your carbohydrate intake. The ketogenic diet eliminates the majority of carbs and replaces them with foods high in fat with moderate amounts of protein. When you reduce the bulk of the carbohydrates from your diet, your body has to rely on fat for energy as oppose to glucose. When your body uses fat as fuel, the body begins to naturally burn fat on its own which helps you lose that extra fat you don't want. So, the answer is that ketosis occurs when you restrict your carbohydrate intake and replace those foods with fats, and a moderate amount of protein. It's also important to not confuse ketosis with the ketosis that occurs with diabetes when the body does not have enough insulin. A ketogenic diet is an intentional approach

13

to entering ketosis, and therefore this diet is dangerous for those who have diabetes since diabetic ketosis is already a risk factor.

You may be wondering how you actually reach ketosis. So, you know that you need to restrict your carbohydrate intake but what else do you need to know about achieving optimal ketosis? The first thing is that reaching this optimal state may take some time, patience, trial, and error. Don't lose hope if you don't reach ketosis your first try. This diet takes patience and adjustments to make it work.

To get started, you will first and foremost want to stick to a very low carbohydrate diet. Start by removing carb heavy items from your diet such as bread, sugar, pasta, rice, potatoes and so on. You will also want to evaluate your protein intake since too much protein can throw your body out of ketosis as well.

The first trick to reaching ketosis is actually to increase your fat intake! I know what you're thinking, increase your fat when you're trying to lose fat? Yes! You need to eat fat to lose fat, and you need to be comfortable with that concept right off the bat. Adding more fat to your diet will help to fill you up faster, keep you full longer and prevent overeating. Fat will also become your new primary source of energy, so it's important to eat enough of it. By eating adequate amounts of fat you provide your body and brain with the energy it needs to function, and it will be easier to enter a state of ketosis. Start by increasing food items such as coconut oil, ghee, avocados, and grass-fed butter.

So, how do you know when you reach ketosis? In order to determine if you have reached a state of ketosis, you will need to measure the number of ketones in your body. There are a few different methods you can use, but the least expensive and most convenient is the finger prick machine that you can pick up at your local pharmacy. To measure the number of ketones in your body, perform the finger stick first thing in the morning before breakfast. The number you are looking for, for optimal ketosis is 0.5-3 mmol/L. Anything higher than three mmol/L is an indication that you are not eating enough food to fuel your body, you do not want to get to this point. The key is to nourish your body with the right foods, not deprive it. Depriving your body will do much more damage than good.

Another easy way to determine if you've reached ketosis is through the breath test. If you notice a fruity smell or taste in your mouth, there is a good chance you are in ketosis. That "keto-breath" does tend to dissipate after a few weeks, so don't worry it's nothing long-term!

There are two methods you can use when first starting your ketogenic diet program. The first method is a low to high method. Start with a low level of new carbs per day, around 20 grams and once you start detecting ketosis, start adding in 5 grams of net carbs per week until you reach a low level of ketones. This is a very quick way to determine what your individual net carb level is.

Another approach to understanding how many carbs you need to reach ketosis is the high to low method. In this method, you will start with a higher amount of net carb around 50 grams and then you keep reducing by 5 net carbs each week until you detect ketones. This is an easier method, but may take a little more time.

Getting into a state of ketosis can be tricky when first starting out, and it may take some time for you to find the right balance. Don't get discouraged, keep trying. Keep playing around with how many carbs you are eating, how much fat's in your diet, and if you are eating enough food for optimal body function. In the coming chapters, I will share a 7-day meal plan featuring the recipes from this book to help you better understand how to prepare your meals to reach ketosis, and remember to be patient and keep trying!

Chapter 4

What's a 'cheat day' and do I need it?

"To keep the body in good health is a duty... otherwise, we shall not be able to keep our mind strong and clear."
- Buddha

Cheat days are something commonly found in nearly every diet program, to help you not feel deprived of all of your favorite foods as you try to lose weight. The question is, what exactly is a cheat day, and do you really need one on a ketogenic diet?

A cheat day on a standard fad diet is commonly an all out binge on things like pizza, cake, brownies, alcohol, ice cream; you name it. Anything you have been depriving yourself of is consumed on a standard cheat day. However, this is not the best idea with the ketogenic diet. All out cheat days can throw your body right out of ketosis.

If you feel like a cheat day, there are things you can do. A cheat day on a ketogenic diet is where you allow yourself an extra amount of carbs on a particular day. You would preferably want to choose slow releasing carbohydrates as opposed to processed and refined carbs. Some items that could be included on a cheat day would be things like sweet potatoes, beans, and nuts. It is also important to know that a cheat day is really only appropriate after you have been on the ketogenic diet for quite some time. Stick to the plan for 1-2 months before you start thinking about a cheat day, as cheat days if done wrong can throw your body out of a state of ketosis.

Do you really need a cheat day? If you can have a cheat day without going totally overboard, then you should be ok. Don't think about cheat days only in terms of carbohydrates either. Maybe you want to eat a little extra cheese with dinner, or amp up your calories for a day; this could be considered a cheat day as well. If you do decide to cheat with your diet choices and add in extra carbs into your diet, do so with slow releasing carbs and only have one cheat meal, don't make it a whole cheat day. Reaching optimal ketosis take a delicate balance and the last thing you want to do is to throw yourself out of ketosis because of your cheat day. After a couple of months of being in ketosis and you want to indulge, stick to one cheat meal and pick up where you left off the next day. Don't let that cheat meal turn into a vicious cycle.

Cheat meals are in place to serve as a way to allow yourself not to feel as deprived and to still enjoy things you really love, but they have to be done right, and they should not be done in your ketogenic diet infancy. Wait until you have some experience with ketosis before trying a cheat meal.

Part 2

The Easy Way to Getting Started

Chapter 5

Tips to simplify your Keto life

"Peace comes from within. Do not seek it without."
- Buddha

Starting any new diet takes some time, and planning which is why I have created a list of tips to help simplify your keto life. Follow these tips to allow for a smooth transition into ketogenic diet living!

Tip #1: Avoid These Foods

- All grains
- Sugar
- Agave syrup
- Ice cream
- Cakes
- Sugary drinks
- Factory-farmed animal products and fish
- All processed foods
- Artificial sweeteners
- Refined fats and oils: Sunflower oil, safflower oil, cottonseed oil, canola oil, soybean oil, grapeseed oil, corn oil, trans fats.
- Sweetened alcoholic beverages
- Tropical fruits: Pineapple, mango, banana, papaya
- Fruit juices
- Dried fruits
- Soy products

Tip #2: Stock up on These Foods

- Grass-fed animal products
- Wild caught fish

- Pasture raised eggs
- Ghee
- Butter
- Coconut oil
- Avocado
- Macadamia nuts
- Olive oil
- Leafy green vegetables
- Celery
- Asparagus
- Cucumbers
- Summer squash
- Coffee
- Tea: Black and herbal
- Mustard
- Bone broth
- Spices
- Mayonnaise
- Kimchi
- Sauerkraut
- Undenatured whey protein

Tip #3: Don't Deprive Yourself

Deprivation is a recipe for dieting disaster. Don't deprive yourself of calories. Your body needs calories to burn fat. Focus on high-quality fats, and a moderate amount of protein to nourish your body and promote energy. If you're hungry, eat! Just eat the right types of foods. Whip up a sliced avocado with a drizzle of olive oil, or make a piece of grilled chicken. Always eat when your body tells you it's hungry. This diet isn't about deprivation, so focus on the foods you can eat and foods like fats and protein that will keep you full longer.

Tip #4: Stay Hydrated

Hydration is critical for overall health. Be sure to start your day with at least 12 ounces of water, and stay hydrated throughout the day, your body needs it. Increase your fluid intake during exercise as well, and add a pinch of sea salt to your gym water bottle to replace essential electrolytes.

Tip #5: Consume Enough Sea Salt

When you follow a low-carb diet, your body needs a little extra sodium, from the right sources. Our kidneys excrete more sodium on a keto diet due to the lower insulin levels. Try adding a teaspoon of Himalayan sea salt into your diet daily, or try some sea veggies such as nori, or kelp to enjoy natural foods high in sodium

Tip #6: Beat Constipation

Constipation can be a huge issue for keto dieters. To remedy this problem consider magnesium supplementation based on doctors approval, and increase your probiotic rich foods such as kimchi, and sauerkraut. Staying hydrated will also help to keep the bowels moving.

Tip #7: Exercise Regularly

Exercise is an important part of a healthy lifestyle and can help you along your keto journey as well. Regular exercise with resistance training and exercise can help balance blood sugar levels and help you reach a state of ketosis.

Follow these tips to help you seamlessly enter into a state of ketosis and start your weight loss journey without stress. This diet takes a little bit of planning, but with these steps, you will be well on your way to keto success.

Chapter 6

What cutlery and gadgets will help?

"As I see it, every day you do one of two things:
build health or produce disease in yourself."
- Adelle Davis

Before you begin your ketogenic journey, it's important to plan what cutlery and gadgets may help make your life just that much easier! Prepping your kitchen for success is one of the key components of being successful in this diet. Here are some of the cutlery and gadgets that may help you reach ketosis, and make this diet simple and fun.

Cutlery:

- Blender
- Food processor
- Skillet
- Immersion blender
- Slow-cooker
- Veggie Spiralizer
- Coffee maker
- Glass Tupperware storage containers
- Hand-held mixer
- Kitchen knives
- Parchment paper
- Baking pans and sheets
- Popsicle molds

Gadgets:

- Ketone body tester: You get a finger prick machine from your local pharmacy.

Pedometer or fitness tracker if you plan to track your exercise.

Part 3
Seamless Keto Dieting

Chapter 7
Common Ketogenic Mistakes

"Never mistake a single mistake with a final mistake."
- F. Scott Fitzgerald

Everyone makes dieting mistakes, especially when you may be unsure as to how to correctly follow the diet guidelines. This is why I have created a list of some of the top ketogenic dieting mistakes to help you prevent making them, and so you can seamlessly start your ketogenic diet.

#1: Eating too Many Carbs

This is more of an obvious one, but one that happens quite frequently when you start eating a ketogenic diet. This occurs more if you don't take the proper steps in determining what your optimal net carb intake is. Once you know that number, it's harder to overeat carbohydrates. Remember to measure the amount of ketones in your body, and as a rough estimate, the number of carbs one should be eating is roughly 20-50 grams per day. However, everyone is different so be sure to follow the low to high or the high to low method to determine how many net carbs your body requires for ketosis. This will be a unique number that works specifically for you.

#2: Eating too Much Protein

Although the ketogenic diet is based on low-carb eating too much protein is not good either! When you eat more protein than your body requires, some of those extra amino acids will turn into glucose. This can throw your body out of ketosis, so don't go overdoing your post workout protein shakes! To be sure you aren't overeating in the protein department, try to stick with 0.7-0.9 grams of protein per

29

pound of body weight and go for 0.9 grams of protein per pound if you are extremely active.

#3: Not Eating Enough Fat

This diet is only effective if you eat the proper amount of fat! Don't be afraid of fat, especially healthy sources such as coconut, olive, and grass fed butter. Your body needs this for energy, now that you are eliminating a large majority of carbohydrate sources. Don't restrict fats or you will be in for some major mood swings, you will constantly feel hungry, and your body will start to break down because it has nothing else to rely on for fuel. Don't damage your body by restricting fats.

#4: Not Being Patient

As we have previously talked about, many people throw in the towel too soon and think that this diet doesn't work. The truth is that ketogenic dieting takes some time, and it certainly takes patience! Play around with your carbohydrate intake, increase fats if needed, and don't be discouraged by those yucky symptoms you may experience the first couple of days starting this diet. Some people quit very early on because they may feel a little under the weather a few days after eliminating many of the carbs from their diet. Be mindful and patient with yourself in knowing that your body is going through a huge adjustment period and just needs time to adapt.

Chapter 8

How to reduce your appetite for sugar and carbs

"He who conquers others is strong; He who conquers himself is mighty."
- Lao Tzu

Sugar cravings are a major issue not just for ketogenic eating, but any diet program. These cravings are often what throw people out of ketosis because they give into them. I have come up with some of the top ways you can reduce your appetite for sugar and carbohydrates so that these foods are a thing of the past for you! With a little persistence you won't even be craving toxic sugar anymore, and ketogenic living will be your new reality.

Step #1: Be Patient

Again, with the patience theme you need to be patient with sugar cravings. Cravings only tend to last an hour or so, and no matter how intense they come on, it's important to remember that they will subside! Give yourself an hour, distract yourself by going for a walk, or calling a friend and you may be surprised to see this craving dissipate.

Step #2: Make Healthier Alternatives

When you're just starting out, it may be hard to kick these cravings overnight, and that's ok. Create healthy alternatives such as the recipes featured in the dessert section of this book. Choose rich foods like avocado to make an avocado pudding instead of indulging in ice cream. Swap in healthier alternative and pretty soon your brain will be wired to crave the healthier version.

Step #3: Eat Frequently

One of the biggest tricks to keeping sugar cravings at bay is to eat regularly. You want to eat small but frequent meals to keep your blood sugar levels stabilized. Your body will feel more satisfied so you won't go into that starvation mode where you want to snack on all the wrong foods.

Step #4: Choose Whole Foods Over Processed Foods

Processed foods are full of artificial junk that can cause food cravings, and blood sugar imbalances. Remove the processed foods from your diet and just eat the real thing! You'll feel more satisfied, and your body will be much more nourished eating this way.

Step #5: Avoid Artificial Sweeteners

Even though artificial sweeteners are often seen in fad diets, they aren't recognized by the body, and your body can't differentiate between artificial sugar and regular sugar. This can lead to sugar cravings. Remove these sweeteners altogether.

Step #6: Take Supplements

Some supplements can help keep sugar cravings at bay. L-glutamine, omega 3's and green tea extract are a couple of commonly used supplements. Remember always to check with your doctor before starting any new supplements.

Step #7: Get Enough Sleep

More often than not, sleep can be the reason you crave sweet. A lack of sleep can cause your hormones to be out of whack and can lead to cravings. Be sure to get quality uninterrupted sleep every single night to promote health and prevent cravings.

Step #8: Exercise

Exercise can help ward off sugar cravings as well. Exercise raises your serotonin levels, just as a sugar binge temporarily would. By exercising regularly, you can keep your serotonin levels up naturally and fill that void without wanting to reach for junk.

Part 4

7-Day Keto Meal Plan

Chapter 9

Quick and easy to do meal plan

"The trouble with always trying to preserve the health of the body is that it is so difficult to do without destroying the health of the mind."
- G.K. Chesterton

	Day 1	Day 2	Day 3	Day 4	Day 5	Day 6	Day 7
Breakfast	Creamy peppermint shake	Berry cream cheese pancakes	Avocado and bacon boats	Decadent cocoa chia pudding	Not your average omelet	Creamy peppermint shake	Berry cream cheese pancakes
Lunch	Veggie taco wrap	Asparagus soup with Greek salad	Tomato and pepper lamb stew	Fresh chicken salad	Avocado salmon wrap	Asparagus soup with Greek salad	Fresh chicken salad
Dinner	Pesto salmon filet	Sweet BBQ pork chops with arugula tomato salad	Spicy garlic shrimp	Zesty Burger with arugula tomato salad	Garlic roasted lamb	Grilled chicken with lime sauce	Coconut chicken
Snacks	Handful of almonds	Hazelnut avocado pudding	Matcha green tea chia pudding	Raw brownie	1 ounce of hard cheese with 8 pitted olives	Nutty Fudge	2 hard-boiled eggs

**Please note that all recipes are located in the following recipe section, and that serving sizes vary depending on weight, activity level, and weight loss goals.

Part 5

40 Mouthwatering Keto Recipes

Chapter 10

Breakfast Recipes

Decadent Cocoa Chia Pudding

This recipe is perfect for all chocolate lovers who don't want to feel guilty after a little chocolate indulgence! This chia pudding has the perfect balance of dark chocolate with a hint of coffee to get your day started on the right foot.

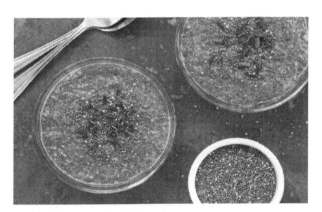

Dietary Label: (GF, V, EF, DF)
Serves: 2
Prep Time: 10 minutes & set overnight
Cook Time: 0 minutes
Ingredients:

- ¼ cup chia seeds
- ½ cup full-fat coconut milk
- 1 tsp. pure vanilla extract
- 1 drop of vanilla crème stevia extract
- 1 tsp. cocoa powder

- 1 Tbsp. Brewed and chilled coffee
- 2 Tbsp. Raw cocoa nibs (1 Tbsp. reserved for topping.)

Directions:

1. The night before you wish to enjoy this breakfast, brew a strong cup of coffee to enjoy, and reserve 1 Tbsp. for the chia pudding, and enjoy the rest of your coffee!
2. After the Tbsp. of coffee has chilled, add the coconut milk, and coffee into a mason jar, or another glass container, and stir. Add in the vanilla, stevia, and cocoa powder, and whisk. At this point you should be drooling over cocoa and coffee aroma! This is how you know your chia pudding is going to be delicious.
3. Add in the chia seeds, and 1 Tbsp. cocoa nibs and stir to combine.
4. That's it! Now, all you need to do is refrigerate this pudding overnight and in the morning you will have magically created an amazing chia pudding breakfast full of healthy fats to get you through your morning. Top with another tablespoon of cocoa nibs in the morning, and enjoy or bring on the go!

Substitutions:

- If you have a coconut allergy, don't worry because you can easily swap in unsweetened rice milk instead! Use the same amount of rice milk to make an allergy-friendly decadent chia pudding.
- If you are not a coffee fan, you can eliminate the brewed coffee, and add an extra tablespoon of coconut milk.

Nutritional Information:

Carbohydrates: 19g
Net Carbs: 8g
Sugar: 2g
Fiber: 11g
Fats: 29g
Protein: 6g
Calories: 344

Creamy Peppermint Breakfast Shake

If you love peppermint patties, but these minty candies are a thing of the past you are going to love this smoothie. Packed with creamy and nourishing ingredients that allow you to have your milkshake and eat it too, even for breakfast!

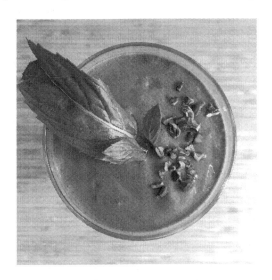

Dietary Label: (GF, V, EF, DF)

Serves: 1
Prep Time: 5 minutes
Cook Time: 0 minutes

Ingredients:

- 1 cup of unsweetened cashew milk
- 1 handful of fresh spinach
- 1 Tbsp. raw cashews
- 2 fresh mint leaves
- 1 tsp. pure vanilla extract
- 2 tsp. raw unsweetened cocoa nibs (1 tsp. reserved for topping)
- 1 scoop of unsweetened whey protein
- 1 handful of ice

Directions:

1. To make this delicious peppermint smoothie, simply add the cashew milk, and cashews to the base of a blender. Next, add in the remaining ingredients, reserving 1 tsp. of the raw cocoa nibs.
2. Now, all you have to do is switch your blender on to blend! Don't be shy here, blend until super smooth.
3. Pour the creamy deliciousness into a large glass, and top with the remaining 1 tsp. of raw cocoa nibs.
4. Enjoy right away!

Substitutions:

- You can use unsweetened coconut milk in place of cashew milk if desired.
- If you love the peppermint flavor, feel free to add in an additional mint lead to enhance the peppermint flavor.

Nutritional Information:

Carbohydrates: 10g
Net Carbs: 8g
Sugar: 3g
Fiber: 2g
Fats: 14g
Protein: 27g
Calories: 261

Berry Cream Cheese Pancakes

If you've missed your weekend pancakes since going low-carb, this recipe is for you! Made without the use of any flour, these pancakes are super decadent and will hit the spot for any pancake lover.

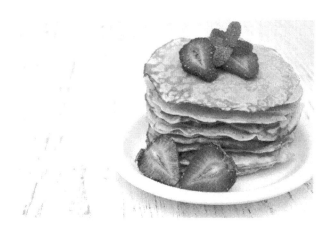

Dietary Label: (GF, EF)
Serves: 4
Prep Time: 5 minutes
Cook Time: 10 minutes
Ingredients:

- ¼ cup cream cheese
- 2 whole eggs
- 1 drop of stevia extract
- ½ tsp. ground nutmeg
- 1 tsp. pure vanilla extract
- 1 Tbsp. coconut oil for cooking
- 1 cup of fresh strawberries, halved

Directions:

1. This recipe really couldn't get any simpler, simply add all of the ingredients into a blender, or food processor and blend until smooth.

2. Next, pour the pancake mixture into a measuring cup and heat a large skillet over medium heat with the coconut oil.
3. Pour ¼ of the batter onto the skillet and wait for these delicious pancakes to be ready. This typically takes about 2 minutes per side. Repeat until all of the pancakes are cooked.
4. Serve with the fresh strawberries and be amazed and how much these resemble real pancakes!

Substitutions:

- If you choose not to use eggs, you can try to use a vegan egg replacer.
- For a dairy free cream cheese substitution, choose a dairy free cream cheese, and use just as you would regular cream cheese.

Nutritional Information:

Carbohydrates: 4g
Net Carbs: 3g
Sugar: 3g
Fiber: 1g
Fats: 11g
Protein: 4g
Calories: 127

Not Your Average Veggie Omelet

If you're tired of the standard breakfast egg omelet, try this spicy loaded omelet to help spice up your breakfast a little.

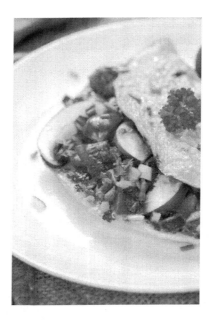

Dietary Label: (GF, DF)
Serves: 1
Prep Time: 5 minutes
Cook Time: 10 minutes
Ingredients:

- 2 whole eggs
- ¼ cup cremini mushrooms
- 1 chopped tomato
- 2 Tbsp. chopped red onion
- ½ jalapeno pepper, chopped
- 1 handful of fresh cilantro
- Salt & Pepper to taste
- 1 Tbsp. coconut oil for cooking

Directions:

1. Simply add the coconut oil into an omelet skillet over medium heat.
2. While the pan is heating, add the eggs to a mixing bowl, and whisk. Pour into the pan.
3. Cook until the eggs begin to cook, and the edges are crispy. Add in the freshly chopped veggies to one side, and fold the other side over to cover.
4. Cook for an additional 2-3 minutes each side.
5. Flip onto a plate and get ready to devour this! Season with salt and pepper if needed.

Substitutions:

- If you choose not to use eggs, you can use tofu.
- For a less spicy option, eliminate the jalapeño pepper.

Nutritional Information:

Carbohydrates: 10g
Net Carbs: 8g
Sugar: 6g
Fiber: 2g
Fats: 22g
Protein: 13g
Calories: 287

Avocado & Bacon Boat

This recipe is for anyone who loves a savory VS. sweet breakfast. Packed with delicious creamy flavors from the avocado with the perfect balance of salty goodness from the bacon. Top this with a fried egg, and you have the perfect breakfast.

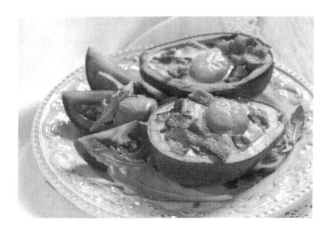

Dietary Label: (GF, DF)
Serves: 1
Prep Time: 5 minutes
Cook Time: 10 minutes
Ingredients:

- 1/2 avocado, pitted
- 2 fried eggs
- 2 slices of bacon
- ½ chopped tomato
- 1 Tbsp. coconut oil for cooking
- 1 small pinch of salt to taste

Directions:

1. After you make your fried eggs according to your liking, it's time to whip up the superstar of this recipe, the bacon. Add the bacon to a preheated pan with the coconut oil and cook until crispy. This may take up to 20 minutes.

2. While the bacon is cooking, slice, and pit the avocado, and top each half with a fried egg. Once the bacon is done, chop into small bites, and add on top of the egg.
3. Season with a small pinch of salt if needed, and serve with a sliced tomato.
4. Enjoy this savory breakfast right away while warm!

Substitutions:

- If you choose not to use eggs, you can sub in tofu.

Nutritional Information:

Carbohydrates: 15g
Net Carbs: 10g
Sugar: 3g
Fiber: 10g
Fats: 47g
Protein: 18g
Calories: 530

Chapter 11

Pork Recipes

Sautéed Rosemary Pork Chops

A delicious herb-infused pork chop recipe perfect for all pork lovers! This recipe combines the perfect combination of garlic, and rosemary for a harmonious balance of pure luxury.

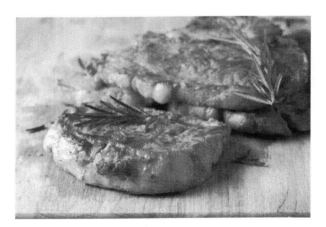

Dietary Label: (GF, EF)
Serves: 4
Prep Time: 5 minutes
Cook Time: 10 minutes

Ingredients:

- 1.5 lbs. pork chops
- 2 Tbsp. butter
- ¼ tsp. cumin

- ½ tsp. garlic powder
- 1 Tbsp. fresh rosemary springs
- 1 tsp. salt
- ½ tsp. pepper
- 1 Tbsp. coconut oil for cooking

Directions:

1. Start by making the delicious pork rub by combining the rosemary, garlic, cumin, salt, and pepper. Rub the pork with the rub to cover completely. Don't skimp on this part!
2. In a large skillet, melt the butter and add the seasoned pork chops. Brown on both sides cooking on high, and then reduce heat to medium and cook for another 5-10 minutes each side or until cooked through.

Serving Suggestion: Enjoy with sautéed vegetables or a side of salad greens.

Substitutions:

- For a dairy-free option, use coconut oil instead of butter for cooking.

Nutritional Information:

Carbohydrates: 1g
Net Carbs: 1g
Sugar: 0g
Fiber: 0g
Fats: 17g
Protein: 29g
Calories: 278

Sweet BBQ Pork Chops

If you're a BBQ lover, these pork chops may be the perfect keto friendly recipe for you. These sweet BBQ Pork Chops are low in carbs, sugar, and bursting with traditional BBQ flavor with a subtle hint of cocoa for a unique flavor.

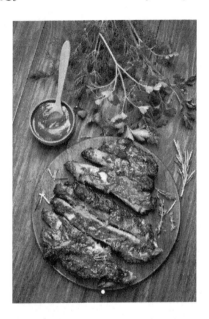

Dietary Label: (GF, EF, DF)
Serves: 4
Prep Time: 10 minutes plus marinate overnight
Cook Time: 75 minutes

Ingredients:

- 1 lb. pork ribs
- ½ white onion, diced
- 2 garlic cloves, chopped
- 1 tsp. paprika
- 2 tsp. raw unsweetened cocoa powder
- ¼ cup olive oil
- ¼ cup no added salt tomato paste

- 1 tsp. cumin
- ½ tsp. salt
- 1 pinch of black pepper
- 1 sprig of fresh rosemary for garnish

Directions:

1. To make these ribs extra tasty, it's best to prep them the night before, so mix up the marinade and let this sit in the fridge for at least 12 hours before cooking.
2. To make this zesty marinade, add all of the seasoning, raw cocoa powder, onion, garlic, olive oil, and tomato paste into a food processor, and blend. Add the pork ribs into a large baking dish, and baste with the homemade BBQ sauce. Set in the fridge overnight.
3. The next day, preheat the oven to 350 degrees F, and place the ribs into the oven, and cook for 1 hour or up to 75 minutes.
4. Garnish with fresh rosemary.

Serving Suggestions: Serve with a side of steamed vegetables, or a side salad.

Substitutions:

- If you prefer a spicier flavor, you can add a pinch of red pepper flakes, or a dash of cayenne pepper to increase the heat.
- For a savorier flavor, try increasing the raw cocoa powder.

Nutritional Information:

Carbohydrates: 6g
Net Carbs: 4g
Sugar: 0g
Fiber: 2g
Fats: 27g
Protein: 14g
Calories: 324

Herb Infused Pork Tenderloin

This herb-infused pork tenderloin is perfect for family gatherings, and is sure to impress. With only a handful of ingredients, you can create the most tender and flavorful low carb tenderloin in under 90 minutes!

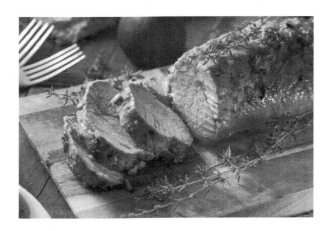

Dietary Label: (GF, EF,)
Serves: 8
Prep Time: 10 minutes plus marinate overnight
Cook Time: 75 minutes

Ingredients:

- (1) 4 lb. pork tenderloin
- 3 Tbsp. olive oil
- 2 garlic cloves, chopped
- ¼ cup chopped white onion
- 4 rosemary sprigs
- 8 thyme sprigs

Sauce

- 2 Tbsp. ghee
- 1 cup low sodium vegetable broth
- 3 tsp. Dijon mustard

- ¼ tsp. salt
- 1 pinch of black pepper

Directions:

1. To make this delicious herb-infused pork roast, start by preheating the oven to 350 degrees F.
2. Add the pork tenderloin roast into a large oven safe baking dish. Rub with the olive oil, and seasoning. Be sure to cover thoroughly! Don't skimp here; you want this roast to be bursting with flavor.
3. Roast the tenderloin for about 60 minutes, or until a thermometer inserted in the middle reads 140-145 degrees F.
4. Once the pork tenderloin is thoroughly cooked, transfer the pork onto a cutting board, and allow it to rest for about 20 minutes. Keep in mind that the temperature will increase as the pork rests.
5. While the pork is resting, mix up the creamy sauce. Add all of the sauce ingredients together in a small stock pot, and stir until melted.
6. Remove the whole herbs from the pork, and pour the sauce over the cooked pork tenderloin.
7. Slice and enjoy!

Serving Suggestions: Serve with oven roasted garlic asparagus, or steamed broccoli.

Substitutions:

- Feel free to add in any of your other favor herbs of choice to alter the flavor according to your taste.
- For a dairy-free option, use vegan butter instead of ghee.

Nutritional Notes:

- Depending on the marinating time, cook time, etc. the amount of marinade consumed will vary. The nutritional information reflects the full amount of each marinate ingredient.

Nutritional Information:

Carbohydrates: 1g
Net Carbs: 1g
Sugar: 0g
Fiber: 0g
Fats: 22g
Protein: 25g
Calories: 304

Chapter 12

Chicken Recipes

Grilled Chicken with Lime Sauce

If you're tired of the traditional grilled chicken breast, this grilled lime chicken breast will blow you away! With just a couple of ingredients, you can spice up the traditional chicken breast to something new and exciting.

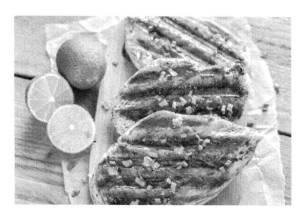

Dietary Label: (GF, EF, DF)
Serves: 4
Prep Time: 10 minutes + 60 minutes marinating time
Cook Time: 15 minutes

Ingredients:

- 4 boneless, skinless chicken breasts
- 1 finely chopped scallion
- 1 garlic clove, chopped
- 3 Tbsp. reduced-sodium soy sauce

- 1 Tbsp. olive oil
- 2 tsp. freshly squeezed lime juice
- ½ Tbsp. honey

Directions:

1. In a large and shallow baking dish, add the lime sauce ingredients: Reduced-sodium soy sauce, olive oil, chopped garlic, freshly squeezed lime juice, and honey. Mix to combine, and add the chicken breast, toss to cover. Place in the refrigerator and marinate for 30-60 minutes.
2. Right before the chicken is finished marinating, preheat a grill outside.
3. Once the chicken has marinated, grill for about 8 minutes each side or until the juices run clear and both sides are browned.
4. Garnish with freshly chopped scallions.
5. That's it! Enjoy right away.

Serving Suggestions: Enjoy with a salad, or alone with some grilled vegetables.

Substitutions:

- Feel free to add in any of your other favor herbs of choice to alter the flavor according to your taste.
- For a dairy-free option, use vegan butter instead of ghee.

Nutritional Notes:

- Depending on the marinating time, cook time, etc. the amount of marinade consumed will vary. The nutritional information reflects the full amount of each marinate ingredient.

Nutritional Information:

Carbohydrates: 3g
Net Carbs: 3g
Sugar: 2g
Fiber: 0g
Fats: 7g
Protein: 27g
Calories: 185

Maple & Mustard Grilled Chicken

A sweet and salty chicken recipe that won't cause you a ton of carbs or sugar! This is a perfect option for summer grilling, and pairs wonderfully with a salad to add a nice protein punch and added flavor.

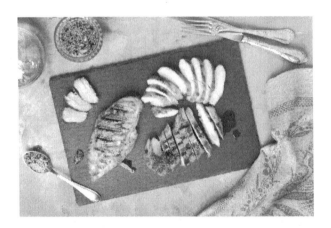

Dietary Label: (GF, EF, DF)
Serves: 4
Prep Time: 10 minutes + 30 minutes marinating time
Cook Time: 15 minutes

Ingredients:

- 4 boneless, skinless chicken breasts
- ¼ cup olive oil
- 3 Tbsp. spicy Dijon mustard
- 3 Tbsp. reduced-sodium soy sauce
- 1 Tbsp. pure maple syrup
- 1 tsp. garlic powder
- 1 tsp. apple cider vinegar
- Fresh cilantro for garnish

Directions:

1. To make the maple marinade, simply add the olive oil, mustard, soy sauce, maple, garlic powder, and apple cider vinegar into a medium sized mixing bowl, and whisk.
2. Next, add the chicken breasts to a glass baking dish, and cover with the maple marinade. Allow this to sit in the fridge for 30 minutes for best results.
3. Preheat the grill, and grill each marinated chicken breast for about 8 minutes each side or until the juices run clear.
4. Garnish with fresh cilantro, and enjoy!

Serving Suggestions: This chicken pairs wonderfully with a salad, and some balsamic dressing.

Substitutions:

- To make this a little extra spicy, add in some red pepper flakes.
- For a vegetarian option, you can use the same marinate for tempeh.

Nutritional Notes:

- Depending on the marinating time, cook time etc. the amount of marinade consumed will vary. The nutritional information reflects the full amount of each marinate ingredient.

Nutritional Information:

Carbohydrates: 5g
Net Carbs: 5g
Sugar: 4g
Fiber: 0g
Fats: 17g
Protein: 27g
Calories: 284

Coconut Chicken

If you love the flavor and texture of breaded chicken, you're going to love this tropical infused chicken breast crisp with shredded coconut for the perfect balance of sweet and savory.

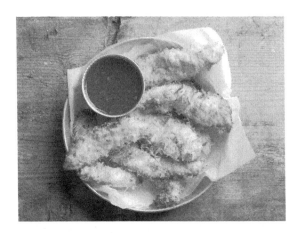

Dietary Label: (GF, DF)
Serves: 4
Prep Time: 30 minutes
Cook Time: 15 minutes

Ingredients:

- 4 boneless, skinless chicken breasts cut into strips
- 2 cups of unsweetened shredded coconut
- 1/4 cup cornstarch
- 3 eggs, beaten
- Pinch of salt & pepper
- 3 Tbsp. Coconut oil for frying

Directions:

1. Start by preheating a large skillet with coconut oil over medium heat.
2. While the pan is heating up, mix the cornstarch, salt, and pepper in a mixing bowl, and set aside. Crack the eggs into a

separate mixing bowl and whisk. In a third bowl, add the shredded coconut.

3. Take the chicken, and dip it into the cornstarch mix followed by the egg mix and finally the shredded coconut.
4. Add to the heated pan, and fry on both sides for about 4-5 minutes or until crispy and cooked through. You will know the chicken is done when the center is no longer pink, and you want the coconut shreds to be crispy and golden brown.
5. Enjoy with a side of hot chili sauce.

Serving Suggestions: Enjoy this coconut chicken tossed in salads or served as an appetizer with a spritz of freshly squeezed lemon or orange juice for a tangy flavor.

Substitutions:

- Use almond flour in place of the coconut shreds for a more traditional breaded chicken.
- Use a vegan egg replacer for the eggs for an egg-free option.

Nutritional Notes:

- Depending on the cook time, the size of the chicken, etc. the amount of coconut oil consumed will vary. The nutritional information reflects the full amount of the coconut oil listed.

Nutritional Information:

Carbohydrates: 14g
Net Carbs: 10g
Sugar: 3g
Fiber: 4g
Fats: 30g
Protein: 31g
Calories: 445

Almond Crusted Chicken

A perfect alternative to traditionally breaded chicken. A delicious low carb option full of rich and savory flavors serving with a spicy dip.

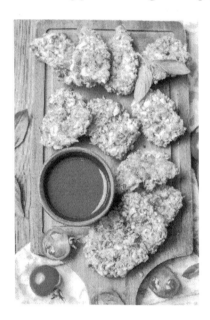

Dietary Label: (GF, DF)
Serves: 6
Prep Time: 30 minutes
Cook Time: 15 minutes

Ingredients:

- 4 boneless, skinless chicken breasts cut in half
- 2 cups of blanched almonds, ground into a fine almond flour
- 3 eggs, beaten
- ¼ tsp. paprika
- Pinch of salt & pepper
- 3 Tbsp. Coconut oil for frying
- ½ cup canned tomatoes, blended
- 2 Tbsp. hot sauce

Directions:

1. Start by preheating a large skillet with coconut oil over medium heat.
2. While the pan is heating up, crack the eggs into a separate mixing bowl and whisk. Add the salt, pepper, and cayenne pepper. In a third bowl, add the homemade almond flour
3. Take the chicken, and dip it into the egg mix and finally the ground almonds.
4. Add to the heated pan, and fry on both sides for about 4-5 minutes or until crispy and cooked through. You will know the chicken is done when the center is no longer pink.
5. While the chicken is cooking, add the canned tomatoes, and hot sauce to a food processor or blender and blend until super smooth.
6. Serve the cooked chicken with the hot tomato sauce.

Serving Suggestions: Enjoy this almond chicken as an appetizer or alongside steamed vegetables.

Substitutions:

- Reduce the amount of hot sauce for a less spicy option.
- Use a vegan egg replacer for the eggs for an egg-free option.

Nutritional Notes:

- Depending on the cook time, the size of the chicken, etc. the amount of coconut oil consumed will vary. The nutritional information reflects the full amount of the coconut oil listed.

Nutritional Information:

Carbohydrates: 11g
Net Carbs: 4g
Sugar: 3g
Fiber: 7g
Fats: 35g
Protein: 31g
Calories: 466

Chapter 13

Fish & Seafood Recipes

Spicy Garlic Shrimp

If you love shrimp scampi, this spicy garlic shrimp recipe takes things to a whole new level! With basil, olive oil, and crushed garlic this recipe slightly resembles a shrimp scampi with a new healthy spin.

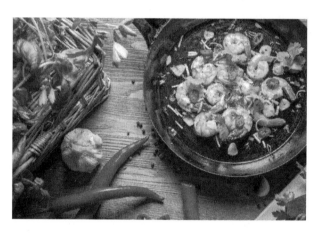

Dietary Label: (SF, GF, DF, EF)
Serves: 3
Prep Time: 15 minutes
Cook Time: 10 minutes
Ingredients:

- 18 deveined large shrimp
- 3 garlic cloves, chopped
- 1 scallion, chopped
- ½ jalapeno pepper, chopped
- 3 Tbsp. olive oil

- 1 Tbsp. ghee
- 1 handful fresh cilantro
- ¼ tsp. sea salt

Directions:

1. To make this new and improved keto shrimp scampi recipe, add the olive oil to a large skillet with the shrimp. Cook until the shrimp turns pink and the tails begin to curl.
2. Add the chopped garlic, scallion, pepper, and ghee. Sauté for another 3-5 minute. Turn off the heat and toss in the cilantro, and ¼ tsp. salt.
3. Enjoy right away!

Serving Suggestions: Enjoy this spicy garlic shrimp with a Spiralized zucchini for a low carb pasta dish.

Substitutions:

- Remove the jalapeno pepper and swap in a bell pepper for a less spicy option.

Nutritional Information:

Carbohydrates: 2g
Net Carbs: 2g
Sugar: 0g
Fiber: 0g
Fats: 18g
Protein: 6g
Calories: 196

Pesto Salmon Filet

A delicious basil infused salmon filet with traditional Italian flavors without the extra carbs! Full of healthy fats to keep you full and full of energy all day, this is the perfect pick me up lunch or dinner recipe.

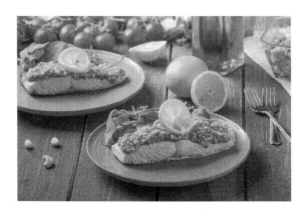

Dietary Label: (SF, GF, DF, EF)
Serves: 4
Prep Time: 20 minutes
Cook Time: 10 minutes

Ingredients:

- 4 (3 ounces) wild caught salmon filets
- 2 Tbsp. freshly squeezed lemon juice
- 2 Tbsp. olive oil
- 1 pinch of salt & pepper
- 2 cups of fresh arugula for serving

Pesto

- ½ cup olive oil
- 2 Tbsp. freshly squeezed lemon juice
- ¼ cup pine nuts
- 1 cup packed basil
- 2 garlic cloves, peeled
- ¼ tsp. sea salt

Directions:

1. To make this delicious Italian-flavored dish start by preheating the oven to 400 degrees F.
2. Rinse the salmon fillet, remove skin if necessary and pat dry. Season with salt and pepper and add to an oven safe baking dish. Drizzle with the olive oil and lemon juice. Bake for 15-30 minutes or until the fish flakes easily with a fork.
3. While the salmon is cooking, make the pesto by adding all of the pesto ingredients to a blender or food processor and blend until smooth. Disrepute evenly among the 4 salmon filets.

Serving Suggestions: Serve with fresh arugula. You can sauté the arugula if desired.

Substitutions:

- Remove the lemon juice from the salmon marinate for a less citrusy flavor.

Nutritional Information:

Carbohydrates: 3g
Net Carbs: 2g
Sugar: 1g
Fiber: 1g
Fats: 43g
Protein: 16g
Calories: 457

Garlic Lemon Scallop

A low carb delicious lemon garlic scallop recipe that pairs wonderfully with sautéed spinach, or steamed broccoli or enjoyed alone. The lemon garlic sauce is a perfect creamy addition to this recipe.

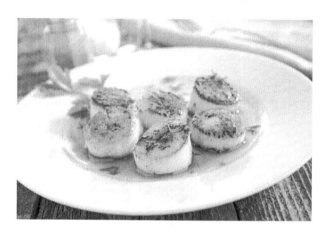

Dietary Label: (SF, GF, EF)
Serves: 6
Prep Time: 20 minutes
Cook Time: 10 minutes

Ingredients:

- 2 pounds of scallops
- ½ cup of butter
- 2 Tbsp. freshly squeezed lemon juice
- 3 garlic cloves, chopped
- ½ tsp. salt
- ¼ tsp. black pepper

Directions:

1. To make this creamy recipe, melt the butter in a large skillet over medium heat and add the garlic. Sauté for 2-3 minutes until there is a delicious garlic aroma. Add the scallops and

cook for about 5-6 minutes each side and then flip. Cook until the scallops are opaque and firm.

2. Place the scallops onto a serving plate, and add the lemon juice, salt, and pepper to the butter mixture. Whisk to combine.

3. Pour the butter garlic sauce over the scallops and split into 6 servings.

Serving Suggestions: Serve alone or with sautéed spinach.

Substitutions:

- Swap out the dairy butter for vegan butter for a dairy free option.

Nutritional Information:

Carbohydrates: 5g
Net Carbs: 5g
Sugar: 0g
Fiber: 0g
Fats: 16g
Protein: 16g
Calories:222

Coconut Shrimp

A low carb recipe that will take you to the tropics! This low-carb coconut shrimp recipe is bursting with coconut flavor and is an excellent appetizer dipped in the chili dipping sauce or served alongside a meal.

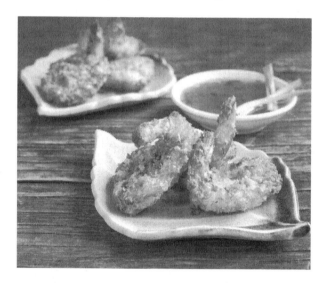

Dietary Label: (SF, GF, DF)
Serves: 6
Prep Time: 20 minutes
Cook Time: 15 minutes

Ingredients:

- 1lb of shrimp peeled and deveined
- 2 eggs, gently whisked
- 1 cup of unsweetened shredded coconut
- 1 Tbsp. coconut flour
- ¼ tsp. salt

Dip:

- ½ cup olive oil
- 2 Tbsp. red wine vinegar
- 1 Tbsp. lime juice
- 1 small red chili diced

Directions:

1. To make this tropical tasting coconut shrimp recipe, preheat the oven to 375 degrees F, and line a baking sheet with parchment paper.
2. While the oven is heating up, add the eggs into a mixing bowl and gently whisk, add the salt. In a separate bowl, add in the unsweetened shredded coconut and the coconut flour in a separate bowl.
3. Dip the shrimp into the coconut flour, then the egg mixture, and finally, the shredded coconut being sure to cover both sides.
4. Evenly distribute onto the baking sheet, and bake for about 15 minutes. Flip over and cook for another 5 minutes.
5. While those tasty shrimp are cooking, whisk up the dip by adding all of the ingredients into a mixing bowl, and whisk.
6. Enjoy the shrimp with the chili dip.

Serving Suggestions: Serve alone with the dip or to accompany a meal.

Substitutions:

- Swap out the egg for a vegan egg for a vegan option.

Nutritional Information:

Carbohydrates: 4g
Net Carbs: 2g
Sugar: 1g
Fiber: 2g
Fats: 25g
Protein: 13g
Calories: 288

Chapter 14

Vegetarian Recipes

Greek Salad

A light and refreshing salad bursting with traditional Greek flavors. This low-carb salad option is perfect for a hot summer day or a light lunch.

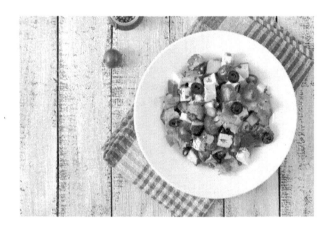

Dietary Label: (GF, DF, EF, V)
Serves: 1
Prep Time: 10 minutes
Cook Time: 5 minutes

Ingredients:

- 1 cup of romaine lettuce
- 8 grape tomatoes, sliced in half
- 4 black olive pitted and sliced
- 4 ounces of tofu, cubed

- 1 Tbsp. of fresh rosemary
- 2 Tbsp. chopped red onion
- 1 Tbsp. olive oil
- 1 Tbsp. coconut oil for cooking

Directions:

1. Start by sautéing the cubed tofu in a medium skillet with coconut oil. Cook for about 5 minutes each side or until browned. You can cook the tofu as you desire. If you prefer it crispy, cook for a few more minutes.
2. Add the lettuce into a large bowl, and top with the tomatoes, olives, red onion, rosemary, and cooked tofu. Drizzle with the olive oil.
3. Enjoy right away!

Serving Suggestions: Serve with a spritz of lemon juice for a citrus flare.

Substitutions:

- Use cilantro or parsley in place of the rosemary if desired.

Nutritional Information:

Carbohydrates: 9g
Net Carbs: 5g
Sugar: 3g
Fiber: 4g
Fats: 36g
Protein: 13g
Calories: 389

Portobello Burger

If you love a good burger and are looking for a hearty and delicious vegetarian option, this is the burger for you! The Portobello mushrooms amazingly resemble hamburger meat. Top it off with traditional burger toppings, and you have yourself a winner.

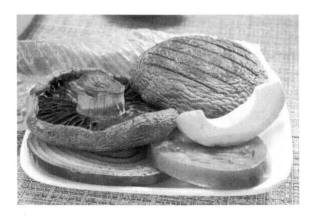

Dietary Label: (GF, DF, EF, V)
Serves: 2
Prep Time: 10 minutes
Cook Time: 10 minutes

Ingredients:

- 2 large Portobello mushroom caps
- 3 Tbsp. balsamic vinegar
- ¼ tsp. salt
- ¼ tsp. black pepper
- 1 Tbsp. coconut oil for cooking

Toppings:

- ½ red onion, sliced
- 1 avocado, pitted and sliced
- 1 plum tomato, sliced
- 2 romaine lettuce leaves

Directions:

1. Start by preheating a grill or a large slotted skillet.
2. Whisk the balsamic vinegar together with the salt and pepper, slice the mushroom stems off, and dip the mushroom caps into the marinade for 2-3 minutes.
3. Grill or sauté with coconut oil for about 5-7 minutes each side.
4. Serve with all the burger goods!
5. Enjoy as you would a traditional burger, but use the lettuce leaf for the bun.

Serving Suggestions: Serve with a side salad, or with steamed vegetables.

Substitutions:

- Add in some heat for a spicier burger if desired. Try adding paprika or cayenne to the balsamic vinegar.

Nutritional Notes:

- Depending on the cook time, the size of the mushrooms, etc. the amount of coconut oil consumed will vary if choose to sauté the mushrooms. The nutritional information reflects the full amount of the coconut oil listed.

Nutritional Information:

Carbohydrates: 17g
Net Carbs: 10g
Sugar: 8g
Fiber: 7g
Fats: 17g
Protein: 4g
Calories: 225

Tofu Southwest Bowl

A delicious traditional southwest bowl vegetarian style! Full of nourishing veggies and a kick of cilantro for a bowl that is bursting with taco flavoring without the carbs.

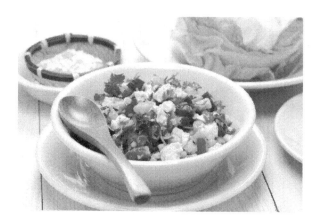

Dietary Label: (GF, DF, EF, V)
Serves: 3
Prep Time: 10 minutes
Cook Time: 10 minutes

Ingredients:

- 2 cups of romaine lettuce, chopped
- ¼ cup of canned corn rinsed and drained
- 1 tomato, chopped
- 1 red bell pepper, chopped
- 4 ounces of crumbled tofu
- 1 Tbsp. olive oil
- ¼ cup fresh cilantro
- 1 tsp. red pepper flakes
- ½ tsp. coriander
- ½ tsp. salt
- ¼ tsp. black pepper
- 1 Tbsp. coconut oil for cooking

Directions:

1. To get started, add the coconut oil into a medium sized skillet and sauté the crumbled tofu for 7-10 minutes.
2. While the tofu is cooking, add the chopped romaine lettuce to the bottom of a large bowl, and top with all the yummy veggies. Add in the seasoning, cilantro, and olive oil. Toss to combine, and top with the cooked tofu.
3. Enjoy warm or chilled.

Serving Suggestions: Serve with lettuce cups for a more traditional "taco" if desired.

Substitutions:

- Swap out the tofu and add in extra vegetables for a soy-free option.

Nutritional Information:

Carbohydrates: 10g
Net Carbs: 6g
Sugar: 4g
Fiber: 4g
Fats: 12g
Protein: 6g
Calories: 156

Chapter 15

Beef & Lamb Recipes

Zesty Burger

A traditional burger with a zesty twist, low carb style! This burger brings flavor and nutrition without the excess carbs. Now you can satisfy your burger cravings without the guilt.

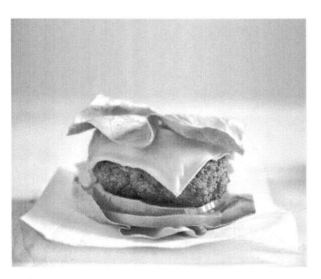

Dietary Label: (GF, DF, EF)
Serves: 4
Prep Time: 10 minutes
Cook Time: 10 minutes

Ingredients:

- 1lb of grass-fed ground beef
- 2 tsp. red pepper flakes
- ¼ tsp. cayenne pepper
- 1 Tbsp. Italian seasoning
- 1 Tbsp. reduced-sodium soy sauce
- ½ cup chopped cilantro

Serving:

- 8 butterhead lettuce leaves
- 1 sliced tomato
- 1 sliced onion
- 4 sliced of American cheese

Directions:

1. Start by preheating the oven to 350 degrees F, and lining a baking sheet with parchment paper.
2. To make this low-carb burger, add all of the burger ingredients into a large mixing bowl, and mix to combine. Form 4 large burger patties, and place on the parchment-lined baking sheet. Bake for 20 minutes, flipping halfway through or until the burger has reached the desired doneness.
3. Serve each burger with 2 lettuce leaves as the "bun" and top with the tomato, onion, and 1 slice of American cheese.

Serving Suggestions: Serve with mustard if desired.

Substitutions:

- Swap out the red pepper flakes and cayenne for a less spicy burger.

Nutritional Information:

Carbohydrates: 7g
Net Carbs: 5g
Sugar: 0g
Fiber: 2g
Fats: 21g
Protein: 26g
Calories: 322

Tomato & Pepper Lamb Stew

A quick and easy lamb stew for a savory dinner packed full of spice. If you love spicy food this recipe is for you, and is packed full of wholesome foods.

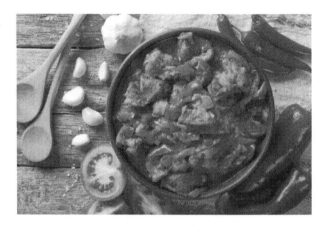

Dietary Label: (GF, DF, EF)
Serves: 5
Prep Time: 10 minutes
Cook Time: 2 hours

Ingredients:

- 3 lbs. boneless lamb cut into 2-inch chunks
- 2 cups beef stock
- 1 red pepper, cut into strips
- 1 red hot pepper, chopped
- 2 tomatoes, chopped
- 3 cloves of garlic, minced
- 1 white onion, chopped
- 1 tsp. salt
- ½ tsp. black pepper
- 1 Tbsp. coconut oil

Directions:

1. To start, add the lamb into a medium skillet with the coconut oil and sauté until brown. Add a slow-cooker with the remaining ingredients.
2. Cook on high for 2 hours. That's it, now all you need to do is wait, and smell the amazing aroma coming from the slow cooker!
3. Split into 5 servings, and enjoy!

Serving Suggestions: Serve with a side of steamed cauliflower or cauliflower rice.

Substitutions:

- Swap out the red hot pepper for a less spicy version.

Nutritional Information:

Carbohydrates: 7g
Net Carbs: 5g
Sugar: 4g
Fiber: 2g
Fats: 24g
Protein: 24g
Calories: 343

Garlic Roasted Lamb

The perfect balance of citrus yet savory this garlic roasted lamb is easy to make and has a hint of lemon with a lot of garlic! If you're a garlic lover, try this roasted lamb recipe.

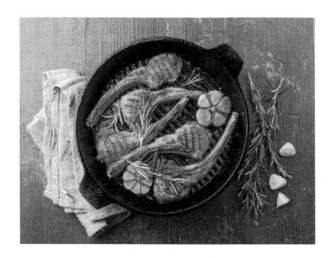

Dietary Label: (GF, DF, EF)
Serves: 4
Prep Time: 10 minutes plus chilling time overnight
Cook Time: 10 minutes

Ingredients:

- 8 lamb chops
- 4 cloves of garlic
- 1 Tbsp. freshly squeezed lemon juice
- 2 Tbsp. olive oil
- 2 tsp. freshly chopped rosemary
- 1 ½ tsp. salt
- 1 tsp. black pepper

Directions:

1. To start, you will want to make the marinade for the lamb chops. Add the garlic, lemon juice, olive oil, rosemary, salt, and pepper into a food processor. Process until smooth, and set aside.
2. Add the lamb chops onto a parchment lined baking sheet, and cover with the marinade, cover and refrigerate overnight.
3. The next day, remove the garlic marinated lamb chops from the fridge, and preheat a broiler. Broil lamb for about 5 minutes each side or until they reach the desired doneness.
4. Serve 3 chops per serving, and enjoy!

Serving Suggestions: Serve with a side of steamed cauliflower or cauliflower rice.

Substitutions:

- Add in any seasoning of choice to adjust the recipe to your liking.

Nutritional Information:

Carbohydrates: 1g
Net Carbs: 1g
Sugar: 0g
Fiber: 0g
Fats: 39g
Protein: 36g
Calories: 511

Chapter 16

Wraps

Turkey Lettuce Wrap

If your keto diet has you missing carbs, don't worry because this turkey lettuce wrap closely resembles the gluten loaded wraps you used to enjoy while packing in health benefits instead!

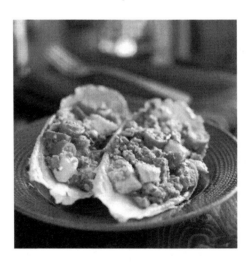

Dietary Label: (GF, DF, EF)
Serves: 4
Prep Time: 15 minutes
Cook Time: 10 minutes

Ingredients:

- 1 lb. of organic ground turkey
- 1 tsp. ground cumin

- 1 tsp. garlic powder
- 1 cup of cherry tomatoes, sliced in half
- 1 cup cubed avocado
- ½ cup of fresh cilantro
- 8 large lettuce leaves for serving
- 1 Tbsp. coconut oil for cooking

Directions:

5. Start by preheating a large skillet over medium heat with the coconut oil. Add in the ground turkey and sauté for about 5-10 minutes or until thoroughly cooked through. Add in the cumin, and garlic powder.
6. Next, add in the remaining ingredients, minus the lettuce leaves and gently stir.
7. Add 2 lettuce leaves per plate, and scoop the turkey mixture onto the lettuce leaf to form a lettuce wrap.
8. Enjoy two wraps per serving!

Serving Suggestions: Serve with a dollop of sour cream or unsweetened plain Greek yogurt for topping.

Substitutions:

- Swap out the cilantro for parsley if desired, and use grass-fed ground beef in place of the turkey if desired.

Nutritional Information:

Carbohydrates: 7g
Net Carbs: 3g
Sugar: 1g
Fiber: 4g
Fats: 11g
Protein: 27g
Calories:226

Asian Fusion Pork Wrap

If you love a good Asian fusion styled wrap, you will love this new low-carb twist. With ginger flavors and freshly chopped veggies, this recipe is bursting with flavor and keeps your carbs low so you can enjoy these wraps without feeling guilty about it.

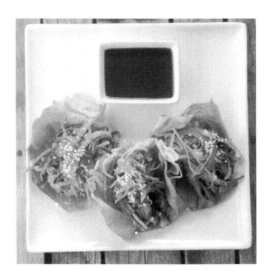

Dietary Label: (GF, DF, EF)
Serves: 2
Prep Time: 20 minutes
Cook Time: 10 minutes

Ingredients:

- 4 large butterhead lettuce leaves
- ½ purple onion, thinly sliced
- 2 scallions, chopped
- ¼ cup thinly sliced carrots
- 1 Tbsp. sesame seeds
- ½ lb. of pork, cut into strips
- 1 Tbsp. coconut oil for cooking

Sauce:

- ¼ cup reduced-sodium soy sauce
- 1 tsp. sesame oil
- 1 tsp. freshly ground ginger

Directions:

1. To start, add the coconut oil into a medium skillet with the sliced pork chops and cook for about 6-8 minutes each side or until cooked through.
2. Add the sliced red onions into the skillet, and sauté until translucent.
3. Add the lettuce leaves onto two separate plates, and fill with the cooked pork, red onions, scallions, and top with the sliced carrots and sesame seed.
4. To make the dipping sauce, simply add all of the sauce ingredients together in a mixing bowl, and whisk. Serve with the Asian fusion lettuce wraps, and enjoy!

Serving Suggestions: Serve with a side of steamed veggies for an added health kick.

Substitutions:

- Swap out the reduced-sodium soy sauce for coconut aminos for a soy-free option.

Nutritional Information:

Carbohydrates: 10g
Net Carbs: 7g
Sugar: 0g
Fiber: 3g
Fats: 21g
Protein: 18g
Calories: 289

Vegetarian Taco Wrap

If you're looking for a way to enjoy tacos without the meat, here is a vegetarian taco wrap that will hit the spot! With a hint of zesty flare, this wrap recipe has the authentic flavors that come with the traditional taco, but formed into a wrap instead.

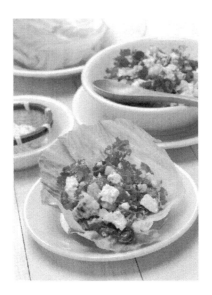

Dietary Label: (GF, DF, EF, V)
Serves: 2
Prep Time: 15 minutes
Cook Time: 10 minutes

Ingredients:

- 4 large butterhead lettuce leaves
- 1 cup of crumbled tofu
- ¼ cup of corn
- 1 hot red pepper, sliced
- 1 handful of fresh cilantro
- 1 Tbsp. coconut oil

Directions:

1. To make this deliciously simple recipe, simply add the coconut oil into a large skillet with the crumbled tofu and cook for about 7 minutes. Add in the corn, and cook for another 2-3 minutes or until the corn is lightly browned.
2. Evenly split the tofu and corn mixture among 4 large lettuce leaves, and top with the hot red pepper, and fresh cilantro.
3. Enjoy!

Serving Suggestions: Serve with a dollop of sour cream.

Substitutions:

- Swap out the red hot pepper for a less spicy version.

Nutritional Information:

Carbohydrates: 8g
Net Carbs: 6g
Sugar: 2g
Fiber: 2g
Fats: 15g
Protein: 14g
Calories: 198

Avocado Salmon Wrap

A unique variation to the standard wrap recipe. This avocado salmon wrap comes packed with healthy fats and omega-3's for a healthy balanced lunch or afternoon snack. This recipe is perfect for salmon lovers!

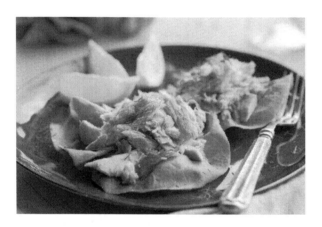

Dietary Label: (GF, DF, EF, SF)
Serves: 2
Prep Time: 15 minutes
Cook Time: 10 minutes

Ingredients:

- 4 large butterhead lettuce leaves
- 3-ounce wild-caught salmon filet
- 1 Tbsp. freshly squeezed lemon juice
- ½ cup cubed avocado
- 2 tsp. fresh dill
- ½ tsp. sea salt
- 1 Tbsp. coconut oil for cooking

Directions:

1. To start, add the coconut oil into a medium skillet with the salmon, and sauté for 7-10 minutes or until cooked through. Season with the sea salt, lemon juice, and dill.

2. Evenly split the salmon mixture among 4 lettuce wraps, and top with freshly sliced avocado.
3. Split into 2 servings and enjoy right away!

Serving Suggestions: Serve with a side of steamed broccoli, or enjoy as a mid-day snack for an added dose of omega-3's and protein.

Substitutions:

- Use tuna in place of the salmon if desired.

Nutritional Information:

Carbohydrates: 5g
Net Carbs: 2g
Sugar: 1g
Fiber: 3g
Fats: 15g
Protein: 10g
Calories: 186

Chapter 17

Side Dishes

Roasted Veggies for Two

A quick and easy side dish for two. These roasted vegetables pair perfectly with just about any dish and make for a perfect healthy addition to pair with a hearty protein.

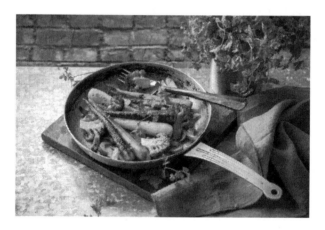

Dietary Label: (GF, DF, EF, V)
Serves: 2
Prep Time: 5 minutes
Cook Time: 5 minutes

Ingredients:

- 4 large rainbow colored carrots
- ½ red onion, thinly sliced
- 1 cup of broccoli florets

- 1 tsp. sea salt
- ½ tsp. black pepper
- 2 Tbsp. coconut oil

Directions:

1. To make this easy and delicious dish, add the coconut oil into a large skillet over medium heat.
2. Wash the carrots, and broccoli and slice the onions and add to the skillet. Sauté for 3-5 minutes until the veggies are brown and the onions are translucent.

Serving Suggestions: Serve alongside any meal. These veggies pair great with baked or roasted chicken or alongside a salmon filet.

Substitutions:

- Add in extra spices and adjust according to your taste.

Nutritional Information:

Carbohydrates: 17g
Net Carbs: 12g
Sugar: 8g
Fiber: 5g
Fats: 14g
Protein: 3g
Calories: 193

Lemon-Roasted Green Beans

A lemony garlic infused green bean dish that pairs perfectly with a flank steak or a grilled chicken dish. Low in carbs but bursting flavor.

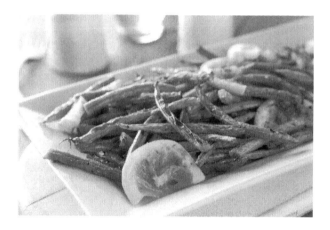

Dietary Label: (GF, EF)
Serves: 2
Prep Time: 5 minutes
Cook Time: 10 minutes

Ingredients:

- 1 bunch of green beans
- 2 Tbsp. freshly squeezed lemon juice
- 2 garlic cloves, chopped
- 1 lemon, quartered
- 1 Tbsp. butter

Directions:

1. Simply bring a large pot of water to a boil, and add in the quartered lemon, and the green beans. Boil for 5 minutes, drain and rinse.
2. Add the butter into a skillet over low heat and add in the cooked green beans, and garlic. Sauté for about 3 minutes.

3. Add the green beans into a serving bowl, and drizzle with the freshly squeezed lemon juice.

Serving Suggestions: Serve with a hamburger, or veggie burger.

Substitutions:

- Swap out the butter for coconut oil for a dairy-free option.

Nutritional Information:

Carbohydrates: 7g

Net Carbs: 5g

Sugar: 0g

Fiber: 2g

Fats: 6g

Protein: 1g

Calories: 78

Cabbage Slaw

A low carb slaw that pair perfectly with a low carb wrap or to serve as an appetizer at your next dinner party. This recipe is truly guilt free, and super light for the hotter summer months.

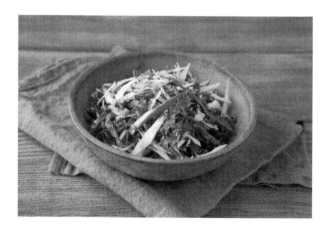

Dietary Label: (GF, EF, DF, V)
Serves: 5
Prep Time: 10 minutes
Cook Time: 0 minutes

Ingredients:

- 1 medium red cabbage thinly sliced
- ½ cup of fresh dill
- ½ of a red onion, thinly sliced
- 2 Tbsp. red wine vinegar
- 1 Tbsp. olive oil
- 1 tsp. sea salt
- 1 tsp. black pepper

Directions:

1. To make this super simple slaw, add all of the ingredients into a mixing bowl, and toss to combine.

2. That's it! You now have yourself a delicious guilt-free appetizer everyone can love!

Serving Suggestions: Serve with a keto style wrap or alongside of a keto style burger or veggie burger.

Substitutions:

- Add in garlic for an added kick.

Nutritional Information:

Carbohydrates: 7g
Net Carbs: 4g
Sugar: 4g
Fiber: 2g
Fats: 3g
Protein: 1g
Calories: 56

Creamed Spinach

If you love creamed spinach, you will love this recipe. This is the perfect dip for veggies, or to serve with a keto style wrap.

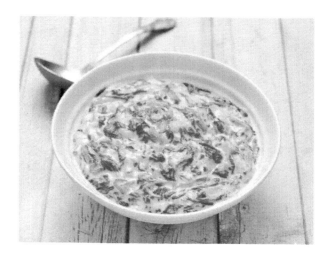

Dietary Label: (GF, EF)
Serves: 10
Prep Time: 5 minutes
Cook Time: 0 minutes

Ingredients:

- 1 cup of fresh spinach
- 1 shallot, chopped
- ½ cup whipped cream cheese
- ½ cup of cottage cheese
- 1 Tbsp. freshly squeeze lime juice
- 2 cloves of garlic, chopped
- 1 tsp. salt
- ½ tsp. black pepper

Directions:

1. This recipe is super easy to make, and only takes about 5 minutes of your time! All you need to do is place all of the ingredients into the base of a food processor, and blend until smooth.
2. Serve right away, or chill for a few hours before serving.
3. Enjoy at your next dinner party for a delicious appetizer!

Serving Suggestions: Serve with chopped veggies or serve as a dip for a keto style wrap.

Substitutions:

- Add in chopped onion for an added kick of flavor.

Nutritional Information:

Carbohydrates: 1g
Net Carbs: 1g
Sugar: 1g
Fiber: 0g
Fats: 4g
Protein: 2g
Calories: 53

Chapter 18

Soups & Salads

Creamy Broccoli Soup

The perfect comfort food, low carb style! This recipe will have you wondering how this could possibly have veggies in it! Super creamy and decadent to hit the spot and pairs perfectly with any main meal.

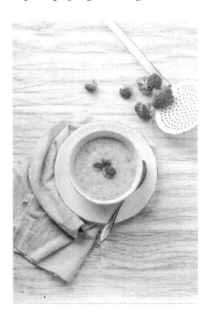

Dietary Label: (GF, EF)
Serves: 4
Prep Time: 10 minutes
Cook Time: 10 minutes

Ingredients:

- 1 head of broccoli, trimmed and chopped
- 3 cups of chicken broth
- 1 cup of heavy cream
- 2 cloves of garlic, chopped
- ¼ cup chopped onion
- 1 cup cubed avocado
- 1 tsp. salt
- ½ tsp. black pepper
- 1 Tbsp. coconut oil

Directions:

1. Start by adding the coconut oil into a large stockpot over medium heat. Add in the onion, and garlic and sauté for 3 minutes. Add in the remaining ingredients minus the avocado and simmer for 5-10 minutes or until the broccoli is tender.
2. Add the avocado into a large food processor or blender, and add in the soup mixture. Blend until super smooth!
3. Enjoy this creamy deliciousness.

Serving Suggestions: Serve with a keto style wrap or alongside any dinner dish.

Substitutions:

- Swap out the avocado if desired, this will just create a less creamy consistency.

Nutritional Information:

Carbohydrates: 17g
Net Carbs: 10g
Sugar: 5g
Fiber: 7g
Fats: 32g
Protein: 7g
Calories: 361

Vegetable Soup

A nourishing veggie soup to bolster the immune system and provide the body with lots of vitamins and minerals. This soup is so yummy you won't even notice how healthy it is!

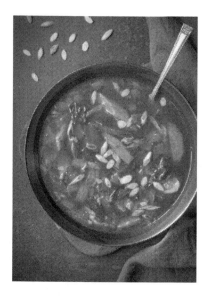

Dietary Label: (GF, EF, DF, V)
Serves: 4
Prep Time: 10 minutes
Cook Time: 10minutes

Ingredients:

- 1 large carrot, chopped
- 1 scallion, chopped
- 1 white onion, finely chopped
- 4 cups of chicken broth
- 1 handful of fresh chopped spinach
- 1 tsp. sea salt
- 1 tsp. black pepper

Directions:

1. This recipe is so easy to make; anyone can throw this together in under 10 minutes! All you need to do is add all of the ingredients into a large stockpot, and bring to a simmer for 10 minutes.
2. That's all there is to it, serve and enjoy!

Serving Suggestions: Serve with a keto style wrap, or enjoy has a nourishing snack.

Substitutions:

- Swap out the spinach for kale if desired.

Nutritional Information:

Carbohydrates: 6g
Net Carbs: 5g
Sugar: 2g
Fiber: 1g
Fats: 1g
Protein: 2g
Calories: 32

Asparagus Bacon Soup

A hearty spin on asparagus soup with a bacon flare! For all you bacon lovers out there, here is a nice way to get in your veggies while still enjoying your bacon. This recipe is super creamy with subtle hints of asparagus.

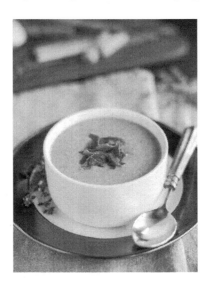

Dietary Label: (GF, EF,)
Serves: 6
Prep Time: 20 minutes
Cook Time: 45 minutes

Ingredients:

- 1 bunch of asparagus
- 4 bacon strips
- ½ of a chopped onion
- 1 Tbsp. coconut oil, melted
- 2 garlic cloves
- 2 cups of chicken broth
- 1 cup of heavy cream
- 1 tsp. sea salt

Directions:

1. To start, preheat the oven to 375 degrees F, and line a baking sheet with parchment paper. Add the asparagus spears and garlic cloves to the sheet and drizzle with the coconut oil. Roast for 12-15 minutes, or until the asparagus is tender.
2. Add all of the ingredients into a stock pot, and simmer for 30-35 minutes.
3. Using an immersion blender, blend until smooth. Season with salt.
4. While the soup is cooking, add the bacon into a skillet and cook until crispy. Crumble once cooked and cooled.
5. Serve the asparagus soup topped with bacon.

Serving Suggestions: Serve with a salad or a keto style wrap.

Substitutions:

- Eliminate the bacon and replace with cheese if desired.

Nutritional Information:

Carbohydrates: 4g
Net Carbs: 3g
Sugar: 2g
Fiber: 1g
Fats: 19g
Protein: 4g
Calories: 195

Fresh Chicken Salad

A light and refreshing salad packed with healthy fats, and protein. This is the perfect complement to any main meal or even serves as an excellent lunch dish.

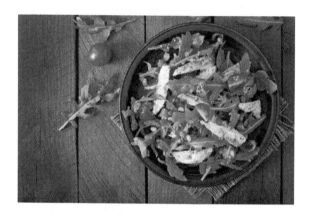

Dietary Label: (GF, EF, DF)
Serves: 2
Prep Time: 10 minutes
Cook Time: 10 minutes

Ingredients:

- 4 cups of arugula
- 8 cherry tomatoes, halved
- 1 chicken breast cut into strips
- 1 tsp. cumin
- ½ tsp red pepper flakes
- 1 Tbsp. olive oil
- 1 Tbsp. freshly squeezed lemon juice
- ½ tsp. black pepper
- 1 Tbsp. coconut oil for cooking

Directions:

1. To start, simply add the coconut oil into a sauté pan over medium heat. Slice the chicken breast into strips, and sauté

until cooked through. Season with cumin, and red pepper flakes and cook for another 2-3 minutes.

2. Next, add the greens into a large mixing bowl, and drizzle with the olive oil and the freshly squeezed lemon juice. Top with the halved cherry tomatoes, and sliced chicken breasts.
3. Split into 2 servings, and enjoy!

Serving Suggestions: Serve with soup, or main dish.

Substitutions:

- Swap out the lemon juice for balsamic vinegar if desired.

Nutritional Information:

Carbohydrates: 5g
Net Carbs: 3g
Sugar: 3g
Fiber: 2g
Fats: 16g
Protein: 15g
Calories: 216

Arugula Tomato Salad

Another light salad to accompany a soup or keto friendly wrap. Light and refreshing and low in carbs with a kick from the red pepper flakes.

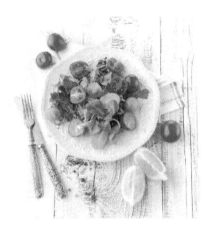

Dietary Label: (GF, EF, DF, V)
Serves: 2
Prep Time: 5 minutes
Cook Time: 0 minutes

Ingredients:

- 4 cups of arugula
- 1 cup of assorted tomatoes, sliced in half
- 2 Tbsp. freshly squeezed lemon juice
- ½ tsp. sea salt
- ¼ tsp. red pepper flakes

Directions:

1. To assemble this simple, refreshing salad, add all of the ingredients minus the lemon juice and seasoning into a large mixing bowl. Toss to combined.
2. Drizzle with lemon juice, and season with salt and red pepper flakes,

3. Split into 2 servings and enjoy!

Serving Suggestions: Serve with a bowl of soup or a keto friendly wrap.

Substitutions:

- Swap out the red pepper flakes for a less spicy option.

Nutritional Information:

Carbohydrates: 6g
Net Carbs: 4g
Sugar: 4g
Fiber: 2g
Fats: 0g
Protein: 2g
Calories: 30

Chapter 19

Dessert Recipes

Coconut Ice Cream Popsicle

You can now have dessert without the guilt while still enjoying all the delicious flavors! These coconut ice cream popsicles are free of refined sugar, creamy and delicious.

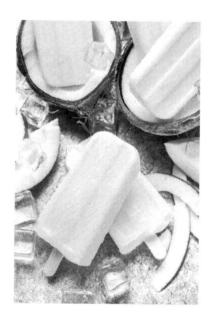

Dietary Label: (GF, EF, DF, V)
Serves: 6
Prep Time: 10 minutes + Chilling time
Cook Time: 0 minutes

Ingredients:

- 2 cups of full-fat coconut milk
- 4 Tbsp. freshly squeezed lemon juice
- ¼ cup shredded coconut

Directions:

1. Simply place all of the ingredients into a blender, and blend until smooth,
2. Transfer into popsicle molds, and freeze for 6 hours or until firm.
3. Enjoy as you would a regular popsicle!

Serving Suggestions: Serve as a refreshing dessert or even as a guilt-free snack!

Substitutions:

- Swap out the lemon juice for lime juice if desired.

Nutritional Information:

Carbohydrates: 6g
Net Carbs: 4g
Sugar: 3g
Fiber: 2g
Fats: 20g
Protein: 2g
Calories: 198

Nutty Fudge

Who doesn't love a good homemade fudge? Now you can have your fudge and eat it too! Rich and decadent and bake free.

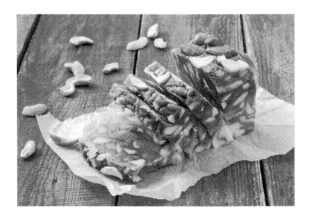

Dietary Label: (GF, EF, DF, V)
Serves: 8
Prep Time: 10 minutes
Cook Time: 5 minutes

Ingredients:

- 1 cup of coconut oil
- ½ cup of peanut butter
- 1 cup of raw cashews
- ¼ cup almonds for topping
- 2 Tbsp. raw cocoa powder
- 1 tsp. pure vanilla extract
- 1 tsp. sea salt

Directions:

1. To make this bake free fudge, add the coconut oil, peanut butter, cocoa powder, vanilla, and sea salt into a saucepan over low heat, and stir until melted. Remove from heat, and add in the raw cashews, stir to combine.

2. Transfer into a parchment lined loaf pan, and top with the almonds.
3. Freeze for 3-4 hours or until firm.
4. Slice and enjoy once hardened, and store leftovers in the freezer.

Serving Suggestions: Serve with a dollop of unsweetened whipped cream for a decadent dessert. (Note this would make this recipe not vegan, or dairy free)

Substitutions:

- Swap out the almonds if desired.

Nutritional Information:

Carbohydrates: 9g
Net Carbs: 7g
Sugar: 1g
Fiber: 2g
Fats: 46g
Protein: 8g
Calories: 454

Hazelnut Avocado Pudding

Finally, a pudding that doesn't come loaded with sugar! This avocado pudding is creamy and resembled that traditional chocolate pudding, so many of us love. This is a fancy pudding naturally flavored with hazelnuts.

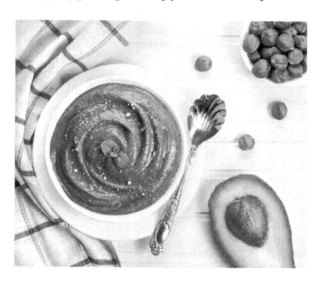

Dietary Label: (GF, EF, DF, V)
Serves: 6
Prep Time: 10 minutes + Chilling time
Cook Time: 0 minutes

Ingredients:

- 4 ripe avocados, pitted and peeled
- ½ cup of unsweetened cocoa powder
- ¼ cup hazelnuts, shell and skin removed
- ½ cup of coconut milk
- 1 tsp. pure vanilla extract

Directions:

1. Simply add all of the ingredients into a food processor, and blend until super smooth.

2. Split among 6 different serving glasses or bowl, and chill for 1-2 hours before serving.
3. Enjoy!

Serving Suggestions: Serve with a dollop of unsweetened whipped cream if desired. (Note this would make this recipe not vegan, or dairy free)

Substitutions:

- Swap out the hazelnuts if desired.

Nutritional Information:

Carbohydrates: 14g
Net Carbs: 5g
Sugar: 0g
Fiber: 9g
Fats: 22g
Protein: 5g
Calories: 245

Matcha Green Tea Chia Pudding

A brand new spin on chia pudding with an even healthier flare! This chia pudding is loaded with antioxidant properties making it the perfect guilt-free dessert.

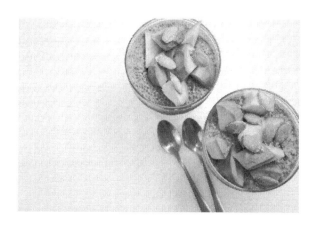

Dietary Label: (GF, EF, DF, V)
Serves: 4
Prep Time: 5 minutes + Chilling time
Cook Time: 0 minutes

Ingredients:

- 1 cup of coconut milk
- ½ cup chia seeds
- ½ tsp. pure vanilla extract
- 1 tsp. matcha green tea powder
- 1 drop of vanilla crème stevia
- 1/2 avocado chopped
- 1 Tbsp. pumpkin seeds

Directions:

1. To make, all you need to do is place the chia seeds, coconut milk, vanilla, stevia, and matcha green tea into a blender, and blend until smooth.

2. Transfer the chia seed mix into a bowl, cover and refrigerate for 4-6 hours or overnight.
3. Split into 4 serving dishes and top with the chopped avocado and pumpkin seeds.

Serving Suggestions: Serve with a dollop of unsweetened whipped cream if desired. (Note this would make this recipe not vegan, or dairy free)

Substitutions:

- Swap out the pumpkin seeds for another nut of choice for topping.

Nutritional Information:

Carbohydrates: 17g
Net Carbs: 5g
Sugar: 2g
Fiber: 12g
Fats: 27g
Protein: 7g
Calories: 317

Raw Brownie

A raw brownie made without flour so you can enjoy a brownie even when living a low carb lifestyle. This recipe is packed full of delicious and nourishing ingredients.

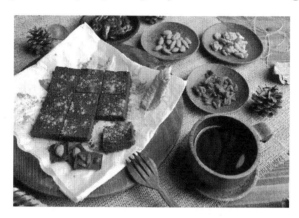

Dietary Label: (GF, EF)
Serves: 16
Prep Time: 15 minutes
Cook Time: 0 minutes

Ingredients:

- 3 cups of raw walnut pieces
- ½ cup of unsweetened cocoa powder
- 4 pitted Medjool dates (Soaked for 20 minutes to soften)
- 2 tsp. pure vanilla extract

Directions:

1. To start, line a large baking sheet with parchment paper.
2. Next, process the walnuts and cocoa powder in a food processor until fine. Add in the soaked pitted Medjool dates. Process until the mixture comes together adding in 1 tsp. of water at a time until the mixture comes together.
3. Flatten the mixture onto the pre-lined baking sheet, and freeze for 4 hours or until hardened.
4. Cut into brownie bars.

Serving Suggestions: Serve with crushed walnuts, goji berries, and almonds if desired. (Note, not reflected in nutritional information)

Substitutions:

- Swap out the pure vanilla extract for peppermint extract for a peppermint flavored brownie.

Nutritional Information:

Carbohydrates: 6g
Net Carbs: 3g
Sugar: 2g
Fiber: 3g
Fats: 15g
Protein: 4g
Calories: 160

Conclusion

Thank you so much for reading my ketogenic diet book! I hope that you have found this book resourceful and that you are excited to get started on your ketogenic diet. I hope that the recipes have inspired you to get into the kitchen and whip up some delicious, and easy recipes that are low in carbs and high in nutritional value.

The ketogenic diet has many perks, and may be the answer for helping assist you in your weight loss goals! Thank you again for taking the time to read my book, and I wish you lots of health and happiness.

Happy keto cooking!

Finally, if you enjoyed this book, then I'd like to ask you for a favor, would you be kind enough to leave an honest review of this book on Amazon? It would help people who are looking for the same information as you to know if this is a book for them or not, and it would be **greatly appreciated!**

Click here to leave a review for this book on Amazon!

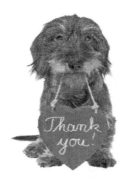

Thank you and good luck!

Resources:

http://ketodietapp.com/Blog/post/2013/11/21/How-Many-Carbs-per-Day-on-Low-Carb-Ketogenic-Diet

http://ketodietapp.com/

http://drjockers.com/10-critical-ketogenic-diet-tips/

http://low-carb-support.com/sugar-cravings-low-carb-diet/

https://authoritynutrition.com/5-most-common-low-carb-mistakes/

https://www.charliefoundation.org/explore-ketogenic-diet/explore-1/introducing-the-diet

http://www.diagnosisdiet.com/ketogenic-diet-safety/

http://www.dietdoctor.com/lose-weight-by-achieving-optimal-ketosis

https://authoritynutrition.com/10-signs-and-symptoms-of-ketosis/

Recipe Index:

Creamed spinach #112
Creamy broccoli soup #114
Vegetable soup #117
Asparagus bacon soup #119
Fresh chicken salad #122
Arugula tomato salad #124
Coconut ice cream popsicles #126
Nutty fudge #128
Hazelnut avocado pudding #130
Matcha green tea chia pudding #132
Raw brownie #134

Made in the USA
Lexington, KY
04 December 2016